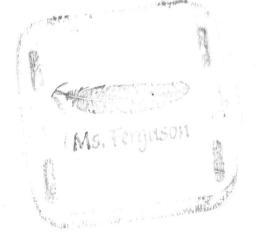

Everything You Need to Know About

YOGA

An Introduction
for Teens

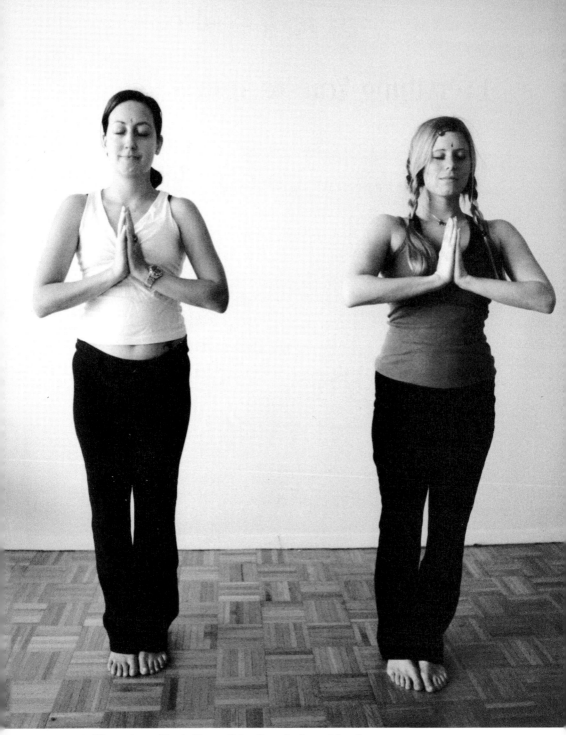

Yoga is a discipline of both mind and body.

Everything You Need to Know About

YOGA
An Introduction for Teens

Stefanie Iris Weiss

THE ROSEN PUBLISHING GROUP, INC.
NEW YORK

To all those on the path: Namaste.

Thanks to all those who provided their wisdom and insight for this project. Special thanks to the models whose perfect *asanas* grace these pages: Adrienne Burke, Christine Rohm, and Matthew Sheehan. Extra special thanks to my friend Kiki Tom, whose photographic expertise made this project possible. Thanks to Sherene Shostak for providing her beautiful space for the shoot. And special thanks to my editor, Erica Smith. Mom, Dad, Hal, Liz G., Nance, Liz S. Ora, Jodi, Miss, Zig, and Caboodle: I love and cherish you. Om Shanti!

Published in 1999 by The Rosen Publishing Group, Inc.
29 East 21st Street, New York, NY 10010

Copyright © 1999 by The Rosen Publishing Group, Inc.

First Edition

Library of Congress Cataloging-in-Publication Data

Weiss, Stefanie Iris.
    Everything you need to know about yoga: an introduction for teens / Stefanie Iris Weiss. — 1st ed.
    p. cm. — (The need to know library)
    Includes bibliographical references and index.
    Summary: Describes the origins and benefits of yoga and provides instructions for performing the basic poses.
    ISBN 0-8239-2959-0
    1. Yoga, Hatha Juvenile literature. [1. Yoga.] I. Title. II. Series.
    RA781.7 .W435 1999
    613.7'046—dc21
                                                                99-30090
                                                                CIP

Manufactured in the United States of America

Contents

Introduction

Lately, the culture of yoga can be seen everywhere. At the 1998 MTV Video Music Awards, Madonna performed a chant while wearing traditional Hindu religious garb. Sting sings on the new record by Krishna Das, a devotee of *bhakti* yoga. On the popular TV show *Dharma & Greg,* Dharma is a yoga instructor. Urban hipsters wear multicolored "bindis" on their foreheads, signaling the expansion of their third eye.

The sudden popularity of yoga makes it seem as if it were invented last week, like any other trend. But the truth is that it's an ancient art.

When most uninitiated Americans think of yoga, they imagine skinny men and women twisted into pretzels. A lot of people think that only hippies and people from California do yoga. They associate yoga with sprouts, antiwar protests, and other "New Age" activities.

In reality, yoga goes far deeper. An ancient Indian sage named Patanjali created a system of yoga, called the Yoga Sutras (*sutra* means thread), more than 5,000 years ago. In it he wrote, *"Yogash Chitta Vritti Nirodah,"* Sanskrit for "Yoga is the cessation of thought-waves in the mind." (Sanskrit is the ancient language of India and the first human language on record. Please note that all of the words that appear in italics in this book are Sanskrit terms. You can look in the Glossary to see how they are pronounced.) The word yoga literally means "union with the divine." When we still the mind, we are better able to access our highest selves. Even the yoga poses *(asanas)* are only a minor part of the practice *(sadhana)* of yoga.

Yoga is an effective pathway to physical health. If you're reading this book simply because you want to find out how to get in shape and look better, you will see that yoga will help tone and shape your body, regulate your hormones, improve your skin and your memory, and increase your resistance to degenerative diseases.

The best part about yoga is that it will make you more beautiful from the inside out. As your appearance improves, yoga will teach you that your body is merely a shell, housing a kind of beauty that cannot be improved upon. Your friends will look at you and notice that you look great, but you will feel great because you know your true self better.

One important note to readers of this book: In many instances the words God, Goddess, divine, soul, or spirit are used. Remember that yoga *is* a spiritual practice. But

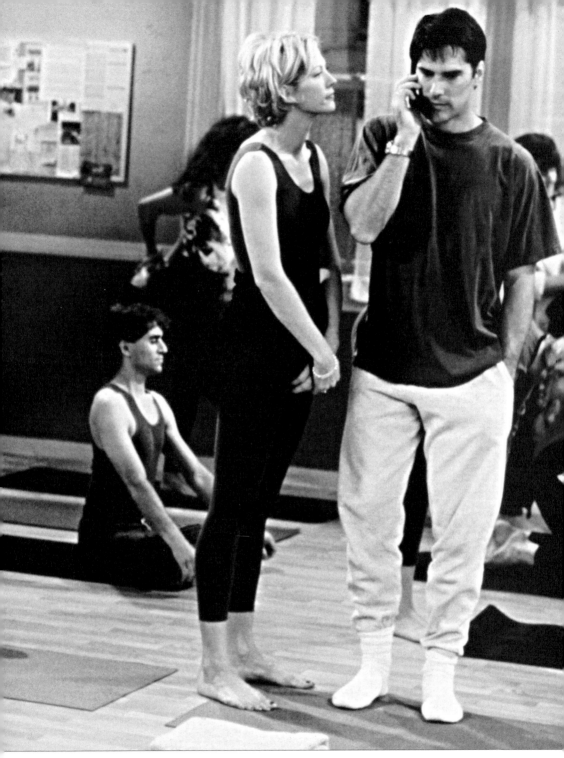

The character of Dharma Finkelstein on the TV show *Dharma & Greg* is a yoga instructor.

that doesn't mean you have to give up your own religion, or worship new deities (gods) to practice yoga. (You might learn some interesting facts about Hinduism, though.) Starting a yoga practice isn't anything like joining a cult. There are Catholic, Muslim, Buddhist, and Jewish yogis! You don't have to renounce anything but hate.

If you have been hearing a whole lot about yoga lately, and you're curious and interested in finding out what it all means, this book is for you. If you want to take a yoga class at the gym or at school or at the local yoga center simply to get fit, you can use this book as an introductory tool. If you want to start practicing on your own at home, the photographs in the book will take you through a series of *asanas*.

Whether you seek relaxation, joy, a healthier body, or even enlightenment, yoga can help show you the way.

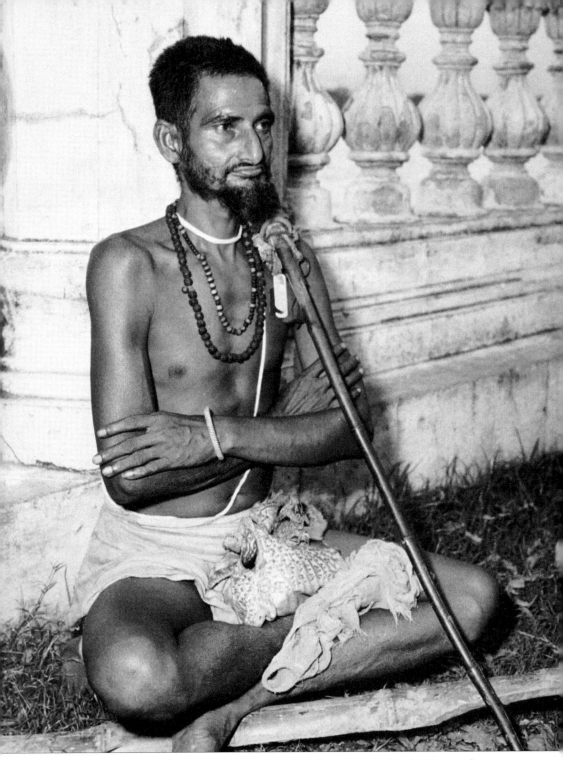

In some parts of the world, the spiritual and physical art of yoga has been practiced for more than 5,000 years. This man is meditating with prayer materials in his lap.

Chapter 1

What Is Yoga?

Indian sages and scientists have been studying yoga for thousands of years. Westerners really just discovered yoga 100 years ago. (Compared to students of yoga in India, we have a long way to go!) Many lifetimes have been dedicated to the path of yoga.

Many Paths, One Source

The word yoga is taken from the Sanskrit root *yuj,* which means to bind, join, and attach. Those who have studied Patanjali's Yoga Sutras loosely interpret this to mean that yoga is the binding of body, mind, and soul. Many modern yogis simply believe that yoga is about learning how to observe what is in the present moment.

The yoga paths can be broadly classified into:

- *Bhakti* Yoga: Path of Devotion (chanting)
- *Karma* Yoga: Path of Selfless Action (activism and service)
- *Jnana* Yoga: Path of Transcendental Knowledge (scholarship)
- *Ashtanga* Yoga: Path of Patanjali (eight-step path)

Patanjali's Yoga Sutras described *ashtanga* yoga, (sometimes referred to as *raja* yoga), or the eight-limbed path of yoga. We don't have room in this book to go into depth about each of these limbs of the tree of yoga, but we will go through a short overview of each limb.

The most important thing to remember about each limb is that it leads to the same place: unification of body, mind, and soul. The limbs, or stages, of *ashtanga* yoga are as follows:

1. *Yamas:* universal moral commandments or self-control; also known as the five restraints.
2. *Niyama:* strict observance of character or self-purification.
3. *Asanas:* body postures.
4. *Pranayama:* breathing exercises or control of *prana* (breath).
5. *Pratyahara:* merging of the senses.
6. *Dharana:* concentration.
7. *Dhyana:* meditation.
8. *Samadhi:* absorption.

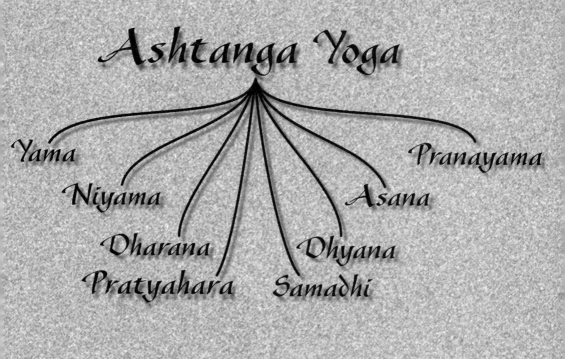

Ashtanga yoga involves an eight-limbed path.

It is very important to have a balanced yoga practice. That is why serious yogis take teacher training courses and read translations of the Yoga Sutras.

Important Concepts
Sadhana
Sadhana is the practice of yoga. Everything you do with the intention of connecting body, mind, and soul is sadhana.

Sadhana can happen around the clock if you let it. Since yoga covers every aspect of life, from the mundane to the ethereal, you never have to give up your practice.

Opening up to it is easy, and unfortunately, letting go of it can be just as easy. But most people find that

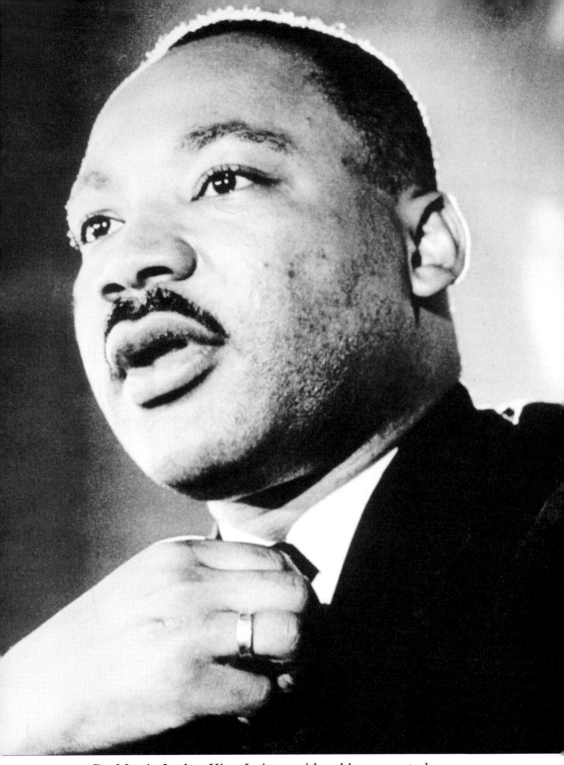

Dr. Martin Luther King Jr. is considered by many to be a *guru*, or spiritual teacher.

starting a yoga practice enriches their daily lives so much that they never want to give it up. Others fight with themselves every time they know they should practice. Learning yoga is a great way to learn discipline.

By picking up this book you have already started your own *sadhana*. Your curiosity about yoga is the first stop on your path. And once you understand the path and practice of yoga, you will be better at everything you choose to do.

The *Guru*

The *guru* is another important part of yoga. In his book *Light on Yoga,* B.K.S. Iyengar defines a *guru* as a "spiritual preceptor, one who illumines the darkness."

A *guru* is really just a teacher. When you read a book by an author whom you admire and connect with, that writer can become one of your *gurus*. If you really like a band and study its lyrics and play its music all the time, the musicians in the band can become *gurus* to you.

In many yoga classes, a chant is sung at the beginning and end of the class that symbolizes gratitude to the *guru*. (I practice at a yoga center in New York City that has an altar strewn with pictures of the Beatles, Martin Luther King Jr., Bob Dylan, many Indian saints, and others. All of these individuals are different kinds of *gurus*.) Many yogis, contemporary and ancient, believe strongly that you cannot search for the *guru*. Instead, when you are ready, the *guru* will appear to you.

Chapter 2

Ahimsa Means Compassion

In the first limb of yoga according to the Sutra, the *yamas,* or five restraints, are kind of like great commandments. They are as follows:

Ahimsa: nonviolence
Satya: truthfulness
Asteya: non-stealing (freedom from craving)
Brahmacharya: abstinence
Aparigraha: nonpossessiveness

The first commandment, *ahimsa,* is the foundation for the rest of the *yamas. Ahimsa,* or nonviolence, is the concept that inspired the nonviolence practiced by Ghandi and later by Martin Luther King Jr.

Ahimsa doesn't just mean nonviolence in the traditional way, not using your fists in anger. To practice

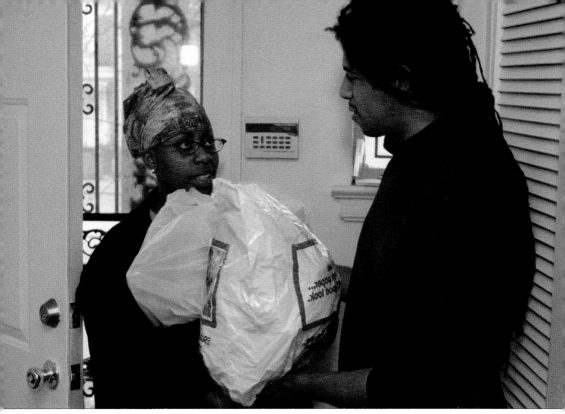

The practice of *ahimsa,* or nonviolence, includes compassion for others, in daily life as well as on a spiritual level.

ahimsa, one must cultivate the *opposite* of violence *all* the time. This is the essence of compassion for all beings. To fully live in *ahimsa,* every thought and action one creates must come from compassion.

When yogis greet each other they say, *"Namaste"* (pronounced NA-ma-stay). It means, "I bow to the divine in you." When you greet strangers with this intention in mind, you are practicing *ahimsa.* You are greeting them with love instead of fear.

You might be thinking, "That's so easy! I'm already pretty compassionate." But *ahimsa* is more than holding the door open for strangers or helping your mom with the groceries or baby-sitting for your little sister—although these are important acts of kindness.

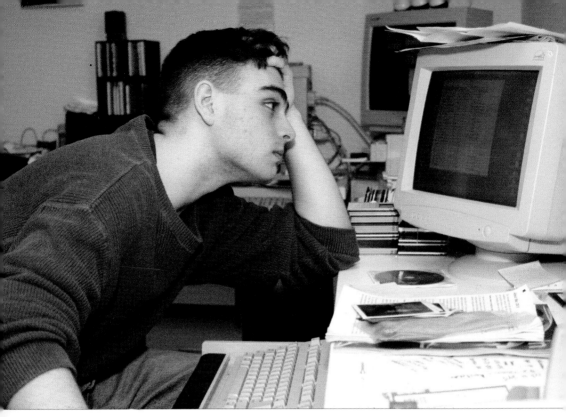

Asanas can help you to relax and cope with stress.

To fully cultivate compassion, one must first love the self completely and without reservation. That's probably why this is the first of the *yamas.*

Ahimsa is at the beginning and end of all yoga. It must stay with you in your practice all the time. Every time we hurt any living being we are not practicing *ahimsa.* That's why vegetarianism and environmentalism are so much a part of the life of many yogis: harming animals is harming the self and the earth. It might sound kind of strange, but one of the basic beliefs of yoga is that all suffering is caused by the misconception that we are all separate. Because everything on earth and in our minds, hearts, and bodies is connected, all of our actions affect other people and things.

Ahimsa is boundless love. We live in a world that sometimes makes it hard for us to access this part of ourselves, the part that loves unconditionally. That is why many believe yoga is currently exploding in popularity in the West—we need it now more than ever. As technology advances, we get busier and busier. Many years ago, people thought that technology would simplify our lives. Instead, faxes and e-mails and cell phones do just the opposite. Sometimes it feels as if our lives will spin out of control. (Relaxation by means of *asanas,* breathing work, and meditation can help.)

Chapter 3

Breathing Easy

Now that we understand the basic philosophy of yoga a little better, let's move on to a study of *pranayama,* or breath control.

Most people usually don't stop to think about breathing unless they get winded. But yogis think a lot about the breath. They do not take it for granted. *Prana* is another word for energy or life force; it also means breath and strength. *Ayama* means length, stretching, or restraint. So *pranayama,* the fourth of Patanjali's eight limbs of yoga, means extension and control of the breath. It is the science of breathing.

If you learn to breathe slowly and deeply, you will in turn learn to live slowly and deeply. Breathing is a metaphor for life.

Katrina was terrified: not only was she taking the SATs in a week, but she had just broken up with her boyfriend, John. Her mother yelled at her from the kitchen as she surfed the Web looking for answers. The screen began to swim before her eyes. Her human relationships were failing, and here she was seeking electronic solace.

She got up and slammed the door to shut out her mother's voice. She sat down in front of the TV to relax. Nothing seemed to work. Everything reminded her of John, and in turn, reminded her that she should really be thinking about schoolwork instead of her ex. All the noise in her life was getting to her. She began to feel as if she were going to have a panic attack.

Finally she shut off the TV and went outside on the porch. She remembered how her English teacher had taught the class some breathing exercises to reduce stress before tests. She closed her eyes and slowly inhaled her breath down into her belly and then let it out evenly.

After about five minutes of controlled breathing, she actually felt better! She couldn't believe it! It was as if her troubles literally melted away in those few minutes. Katrina went back inside and sat back down at her computer. Instead of surfing the Web or going to a chat room to escape the pressure of her life, she booted up her SAT program. She had the best study session yet.

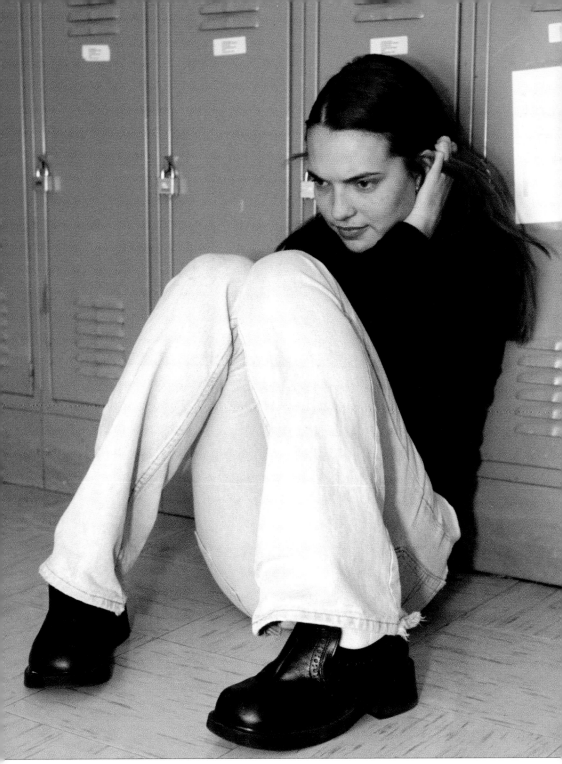

When you are tense, deep breathing can really calm you down.

Katrina used breath work to regain control of a stressful situation. She may not have known that the breathing exercise she chose to do was also the ancient science of *pranayama*.

Breath Is Your Friend

It is very important for the beginning yogi to honor his or her own style of breathing. You might not have thought that your breathing had a "style," but it does.

Your first task is to become friends with your breath. While you are sitting in class or at the kitchen table, stop for a moment and just listen to your breath. Remember that breath is already a constant companion; it has been with you since the moment you were born and will be with you until you "leave your body." (This is how yogis describe physical death.)

When we get to the chapter on *asanas* you will see how integral the breath is to the practice of yoga. In yoga, all breath is inhaled and exhaled through the nose. Yoga teachers stress the importance of coming back to the breath no matter where one is in their practice. You go as far as you can in a pose, and then just "be with the breath." Even if you can't get your legs over your head, for instance, just stop where you are (before it hurts) and breathe. It's that simple.

The advanced exercises that you might read about in other books should only be undertaken after you have studied yoga for a long time. We are concentrating here on using breath correctly while performing the *asanas* and remembering the importance of the breath in daily life. You must do much *sadhana* and study for quite a while before you can do the more advanced exercises.

But even when you first start your *sadhana,* you can learn to count your breaths and slow them down. This will impart a deep peacefulness to you and help you to eventually avoid the syndrome of becoming "out of breath."

Good yoga teachers will always help you perfect the science of breath. They will guide you through the breath as it relates to the *asanas.* While doing *asana* practice, you breathe only through the nose. The slow, controlled, audible breathing done during *asana* practice is called *ujayii* (YOU-jie) breath. There is an opening between the vocal cords called the glottis. Try to partially close this and breathe slowly in and out through the nose. Try to make a smooth sound as you exhale.

Mulabhanda

If you plan to start practicing yoga on your own, you must also learn to control *mulabhanda. Mula* means "root." *Bhanda* means "to hold or contract." So, to perfect *mulabhanda* is to learn to "hold the root" of your body.

To apply *mulabhanda,* simply contract the muscles in the anus to the belly button and try to imagine lifting that part of your body to your spine. This promotes strong stomach muscles. You should apply *mulabhanda* in almost every *asana.*

Don't get frustrated by how difficult it seems at first to control *mulabhanda*. It takes a long time to perfect—be patient with yourself. Often if we imagine our bodies moving in a certain way, our muscles will react involuntarily and obey our minds.

Let's begin to explore the *asanas* and start to deepen our practice.

Chapter 4

Strike a Pose

Now you're ready to begin your *asana* practice. The most important thing to remember at first is that wherever you are, that's where you're supposed to be. Never, under any circumstance, should you experience pain or strain in an *asana*. If you are practicing in a group, try to keep your focus on your own postures and breathing, and not on the technique of the person next to you.

Don't get caught up in being "good" at yoga. The only person you are competing with is you. Go at your own pace.

This section is directed toward those who will begin their practice alone. But many of the rules apply to those in a group as well. It is recommended that, whenever possible, the new yogi should find a teacher/*guru* to work with. Your teacher can align you when you're not fully in a pose and help you in a thousand other ways.

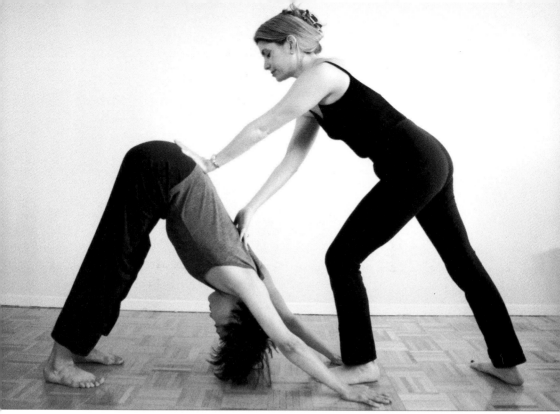

A *guru* or teacher can help you to reach your yoga pose.

Please read through the entire book before you start practicing. Study the photographs. Maybe even go to the video store or the library and browse the yoga videos. (Consult the listings in the Where to Go for Help section for ideas.)

Where to Practice

First, find a clean, quiet space in your home where you can have some privacy. Try to practice on a level floor. Make sure there is room overhead for you to raise your arms as high as they can go. Make sure the room is well heated. Do not practice in direct sunlight. Wear loose, comfortable clothing. Take off your shoes and socks. You can put on some music if you want. Make sure it

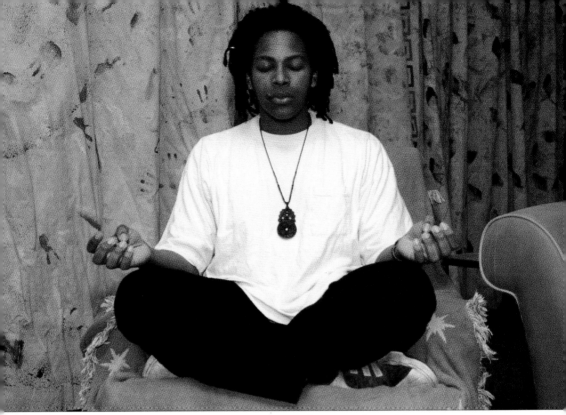

Find a quiet, private spot to practice your breathing.

is playing softly enough so that you can hear yourself breathe. (There are some suggestions for audio and video selections at the end of the book. It's a great idea to use a video at first for some guidance.)

When to Practice

Always practice on an empty stomach. Wait three or four hours after you have eaten a full meal, or at least one hour after eating a light meal. The best time to practice is in the early morning, before you have had anything to eat.

How Long to Practice

It's best to practice every day, so if you can only fit in a half an hour on some days, that's enough. Even a five-minute yoga session in the morning will enrich your day.

The lesson in this book should take you about forty-five minutes. The ideal length of practice is two or three hours for advanced students.

Tools

A nonslip surface (like a hardwood or linoleum floor or a firm rug) is the best for practice. One of the most important pieces of equipment for yoga is the "sticky mat." (Places where these mats can be purchased are listed in the Where to Go for Help section at the end of the book.) Try to avoid practicing on a rug that is not firmly tacked to the ground. This will make your practice difficult.

A note to girls: As a rule, do not practice when you have your period. After the third day of bleeding, some teachers believe you can begin a light practice again, but never do any inversions while you are bleeding. (Inversions include the shoulder stand, headstand, handstand, and others.) If you are working with a teacher, however, he or she can show you several postures that are actually beneficial for you during your period. They can alleviate cramps and regulate the cycle. We'll go over some of them in a later chapter.

Most women can practice yoga while pregnant, almost up until the time of birth. But there are certain poses that are dangerous to the developing fetus. Many yoga centers offer prenatal yoga classes. It is recommended that pregnant women consult their doctors before taking up new practices or continuing to practice yoga.

Prepare to sweat! Keep a towel handy in case you get too slippery. But remember that sweating is a good sign. It means that you are warmed up, working hard, and burning energy. That's what you're supposed to do! You might be pretty sore the next day, but it will be a good kind of sore, the kind that reminds you of all the hard work you've done. Remember, don't forget to breathe!

"Om"

Most yoga classes begin with chanting of the word "om." "Om" is the universal, primordial sound. It is represented by a symbol. (One of the reasons that it is helpful to watch a video or attend a yoga class is that you will be instructed in the proper way to chant. We will discuss chanting further in chapter 6.) It is sung slowly, usually three times, at three different pitches. The eyes should be closed and you should sit either cross-legged or in the Lotus position. (This is the pose most people associate with yoga. You've probably seen pictures of people in this pose before.) Just stick with whatever is more comfortable.

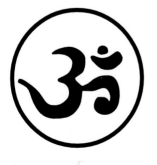

Lotus Pose is also called *Padmasana.* Sit on the floor. Rest your hands on your knees, with palms facing up if you want. Raise the left foot up onto the right thigh, as close to the hip as possible. Do the same with the left foot on the right thigh.

This is the symbol for Om.

Close your eyes and take a deep breath. Chant the word "om" pronouncing each part of the word as long and deep as you can: "A-U-M." Do this three times. This *asana* is the basic meditation *asana,* so we really start each *asana* practice with a brief meditation. Breathe deeply. Open your eyes. Bring your awareness to any part of your body that feels out of sorts. Think about how the *asana* practice you are about to do will heal that pain.

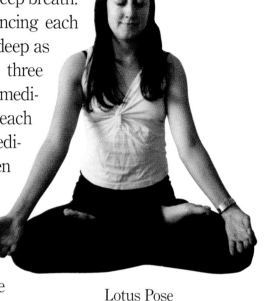

Lotus Pose

Poses
Sun Salutation

Now we are ready for the Sun Salutation, or *Surya Namaskara A.* The Sun Salutation is done 180 times every morning at sunrise by yogis in India. (Don't worry—we're going to start with only five.) This first pose is the foundation of your *asana* practice. You will always come back to it. Learn it and love it with all your heart.

It might sound easy at first, but it really takes time to perfect. When you embody that perfection for the first time, you will feel blissful. The first time you go through the various poses in the Sun Salutation, spend a few moments in each one and feel it well. After you

feel more comfortable with each position, you can begin
to do the Sun Salutation as a flowing series of poses.
The Sun Salutation is a kind of warm-up. When you are
finished you should be sweating a bit. The name of the
first *asana* in the Sun Salutation is *Samastihiti* (sah-
MAH-stee-ha-tee).

1. Equal Standing Pose, or *Samastihiti:* Stand up
straight, with your heels and big toes touching and your
arms at your side. Imagine your body as a stake driven
into the earth. Connect to the ground with the soles of
your feet. Balance. Make sure your spine is erect and
your weight is distributed equally between your heels
and toes. Stand perfectly still and breathe. Apply *mulabhanda.* The eyes should remain steady on a point in
front of you. **(Photo 1)**

2. Inhaling, raise your arms above your head, placing
the palms together at the end of the breath. Look at
your thumbs. **(Photo 2)**

3. Exhaling, bend forward and pull back the pubic
bone in time with the breath. Point the top of the head
straight down toward the toes. Place the hands on the
floor beside the feet, if possible. This might be hard for
you at first. Most people can't touch their toes when
they first start their *asana* practice, but that's okay. Just
go as far as you can without straining. **(Photo 3)**

4. Inhaling, lift the head and rise to a flat back, as if
you were making a table out of your body. Keep the tips
of the fingers on the floor, if you can. **(Photo 4)**

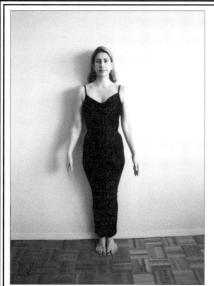

Photo 1

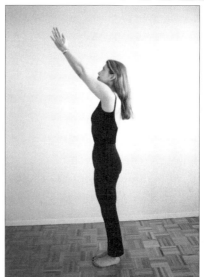

Photo 2

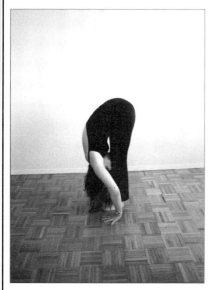

Photo 3

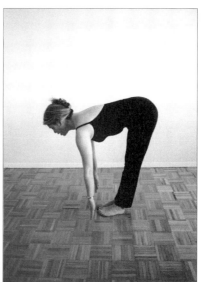

Photo 4

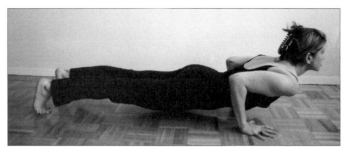

Photo 5

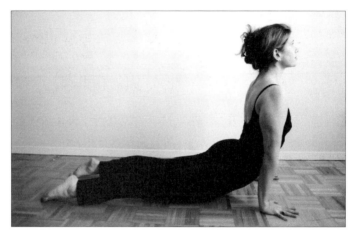

Photo 6

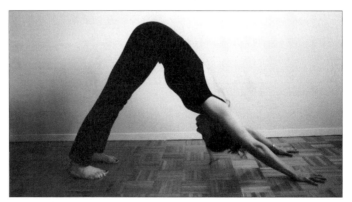

Photo 7

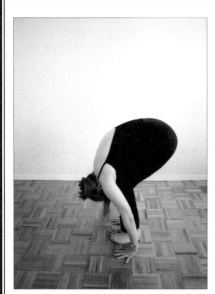

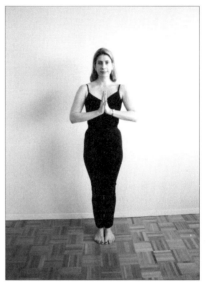

Photo 8   Photo 9

5. Exhaling, step back and separate the feet to hip width. (Once you have practiced for some time you will hop back into the next pose.) Try to lower the body until it is two to four inches from the floor. Keep the shoulders squared and elbows close to the sides. This is called *Chaturanga Dandasana.* **(Photo 5)**

6. Inhaling, come forward and up, pointing the toes. Arch the back and rest on the hands. Straighten your arms and lift your heart. This *asana* is called Upward Facing Dog, or *Urdhva Mukha Svanasana.* It takes a while to master moving from *Chaturanga* to Upward Facing Dog. The idea is to avoid putting your belly on the floor as you move into the next pose. Rely on your arm strength. **(Photo 6)**

7. Exhaling, pull back your groin, roll over your toes, and come into Downward Facing Dog, or *Adho Mukha Svanasana*. Make sure your fingers and toes spread wide and are pushing down into the ground. Draw your butt up toward the ceiling. Press your heels into the floor. Look toward your belly button. Stay for five breaths. **(Photo 7)**

8. With the second part of your last breath, look at the floor between your hands and step between the hands, first with one foot and then the other. (After some time you will learn to hop back into the next pose.) As you lift your feet, raise your head and look between your eyebrows, making your back flat again. **(Photo 8)**

9. Exhale and fold to your legs, bringing your face as close as possible to your knees. This is just like photo 3 or description number 3.

10. Exhale and return to Equal Standing Pose. If you want, you can bring your hands together in front of your heart in prayer position. **(Photo 9)** You can also take this moment to repeat your *mantra*. (See chapter six.) Take a few breaths and clear the mind.

The Sun Salutation promotes coordination and stability. It should be done a minimum of three times. Before you begin to experiment with other poses, it is recommended that you become very comfortable with the Sun Salutation.

Warrior Pose
The next pose we will explore is called Warrior Pose or *Virabhadrasana A*.

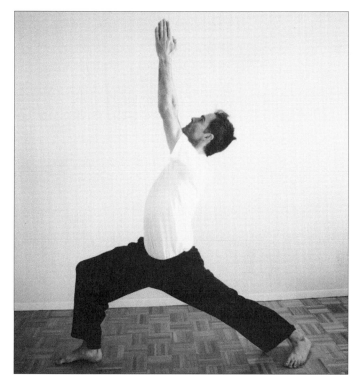

Warrior Pose 1

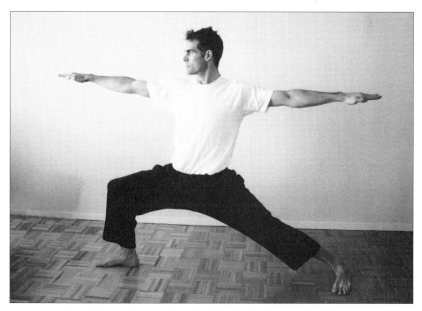

Warrior Pose 2

1. Stand in *Samastihiti*. Take a deep breath and jump so that your feet are spread about four feet wide. Turn so that your right foot faces the right wall at a ninety-degree angle and your left foot is at a diagonal, also in the direction of the right wall. Exhale. Bend your right knee and try to lower it until it goes over your right ankle. Keep both of your feet firmly grounded. Lift your arms over your head, palms touching, and look at your thumbs. Open the heart. Breathe five breaths.

2. Step back into Equal Standing Pose and breathe, and then do the pose on the left side. Or, as an alternative, pivot on the heels and do the same on the left side without pausing in Equal Standing Pose.

Next we will do Warrior 2:

1. Go into Warrior 1 on the right side. Before you take your five breaths, open your arms wide and spread your right arm in front of you and your left arm behind you, as if two people were pulling you from either side. Gaze at the right palm. Now take five breaths. Reverse your position and do the same on the left side.

2. Inhale and jump back to *Samastihiti*. This pose is excellent for the legs. It makes you stronger and better able to do advanced poses.

Triangle Pose (*Trikonasana*)

1. Stand in Equal Standing Pose. Inhale deeply and jump to spread the legs apart about three feet. Raise

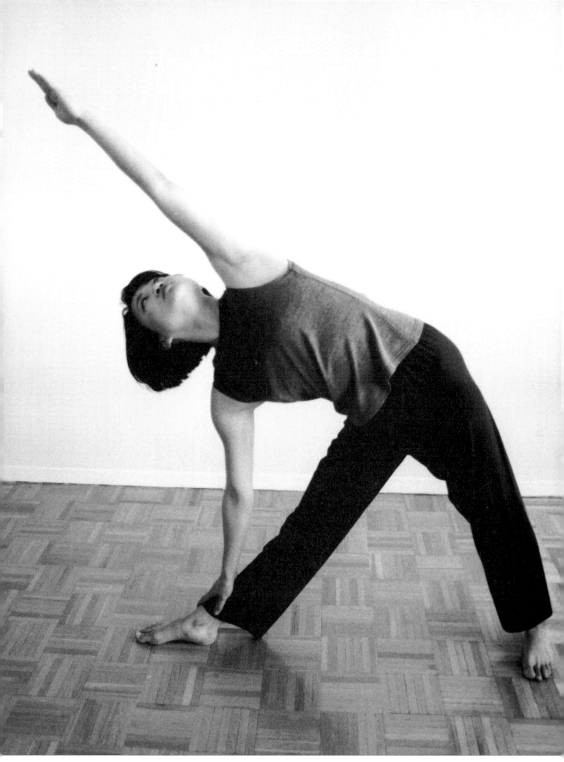

Triangle Pose

the arms sideways in line with the shoulders, palms facing down.

2. Turn the right foot sideways and ninety degrees to the right. Turn the left foot slightly to the right (on a diagonal).

3. Exhale and bend the torso sideways to the right, bringing the right palm close to the right ankle, on the outside of the foot. If you can't reach the floor, grab whatever part of your leg you can reach. Reach the left arm up and bring it in line with the right shoulder. Look up at your thumb. Stay for five breaths.

4. Lower your arms and pivot to the left. Repeat on the left side.

This pose can relieve backaches and neck sprains. It also tones and strengthens the legs.

Child's Pose *(Balakasana)*

Now let's look at a resting pose. This *asana* is called Child's Pose or *Balakasana.* Whenever you are feeling tired, or if a pose has strained you for any reason, stop and rest for a few breaths in Child's Pose. This pose is thought to increase memory and strengthen eyesight.

Simply kneel down on your knees and sit back on your calves comfortably. Inhale a breath, and raise your arms above your head. Bend forward so that your head touches the ground in front of your knees.

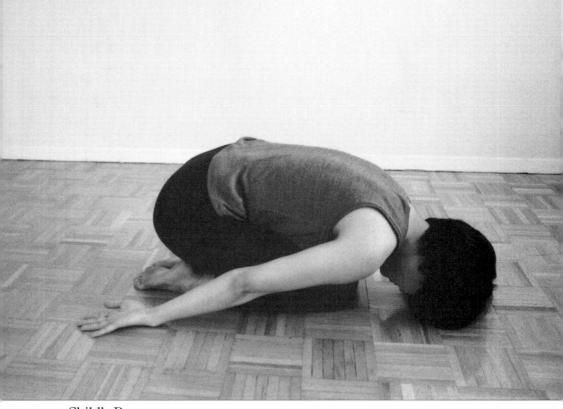

Child's Pose

Exhale. Your hands can stretch beyond your knees in front of you, or back behind you next to your thighs, palms facing up. Rest and breathe here as long as you need to.

Relaxation Pose *(Shavasana)*
The final pose in our *asana* series is Relaxation Pose, or *Shavasana.* Final Relaxation, or Corpse Pose, as it's sometimes called, should be done at the end of each practice. It recharges, relieves fatigue, and reduces stress. You might want to dim the lights and cover yourself with a blanket for this pose to make it more cozy. As much as possible, try to free your mind from any thoughts.

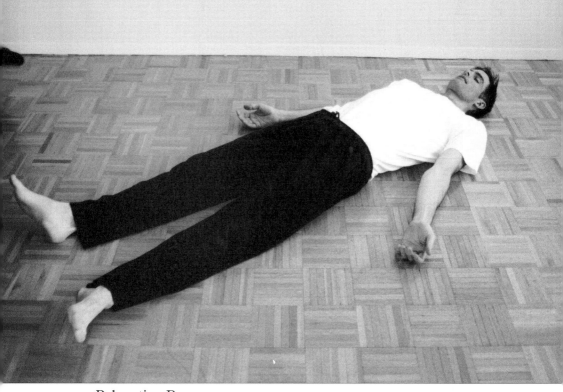
Relaxation Pose

Try not to fall asleep for more than the time you have designated for the pose. If you want to sleep, go to your bed or the couch so that your yoga space and your sleeping space remain separate.

Lie flat on the back, arms at the sides and head relaxed. Close your eyes and relax, breathing normally. This should be done for about ten minutes.

There are many other *asanas* that you can experiment with. You can add some of the options from the next chapter if they are appealing to you. Be creative! Once again, it will help a lot if you check out some yoga videos or go to a class.

Chapter 5

Curing What Ails You

Now we have learned many of the ways that yoga can heal your life. Maybe you already feel better just from starting your quest. The seeker sees the truth much clearer once he or she sets on the path. But let's look specifically at some of the physical discomfort for which you might seek relief.

Premenstrual Syndrome (PMS)

Most girls experience PMS and cramping during their period. The pain can be overwhelming. Who can concentrate on homework or life in general when she is having a bad period? It's not easy. But yoga can help alleviate some of that pain.

Nobility Pose *(Bhadrasana)*

Do your periods come too late or too early? Are they

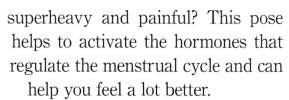

Nobility Pose

superheavy and painful? This pose helps to activate the hormones that regulate the menstrual cycle and can help you feel a lot better.

Sit on the floor and bring the soles of the feet together. Close the eyes. Clasp the hands around the feet, and pull the heels as close in to the body as possible. Inhale slowly and try to keep the head, spine, and neck in a straight line. Push the knees to the floor. Hold your breath in at a comfortable level for five counts. Exhale. (This can also be used as a meditation pose, breathing normally.)

Cat Pose *(Vidalasana)*
The next pose helps digestion and is also recommended during menstruation.

1. Kneel on all fours, with hands and knees slightly apart. Make sure your arms and thighs are perpendicular to the floor. Make the mouth like a pipe and inhale through it with a hissing sound. (This is an exception to the rule of nose-only breathing during *asana* practice.) At the same time, round the back up like a cat and lower the head. Hold the breath for a few moments in this position.

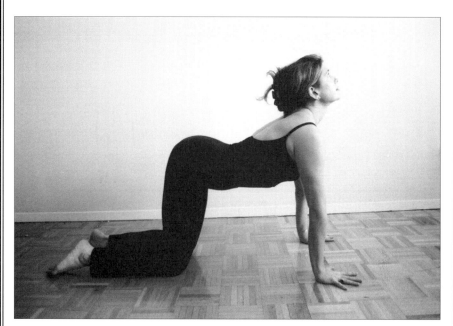

Cat Pose

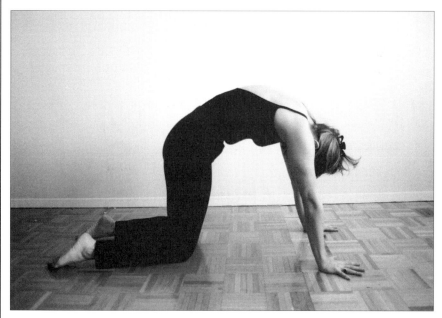

Cat Pose

2. Exhale slowly through the mouth, arching the back in and moving your belly toward the floor. Look up. Do this pose several times.

Headaches

Another common ailment of teenagers is headaches. We get headaches for lots of different reasons. Sometimes stress or hunger can cause a headache. When a headache results from stress, it often originates in the neck. This kind of headache can be treated with the following poses:

> Mountain Pose, or *Tadasana,* is a great headache cure. It sometimes helps to use a wall when you are using *Tadasana* for a headache; the wall makes it easier to align the spine.

> Downward Facing Dog is also helpful for headaches. The weight of the head will stretch the neck.

Asthma

The pose *Uttanasana* is useful for asthmatics. It is also said to be helpful for depression, menstrual irregularity, and nervous tension.

1. Stand in Mountain Pose. Exhale, bend forward, and place your hands on the floor next to or just behind your feet, if you can reach. If you can't reach, just hang there as low as you can.

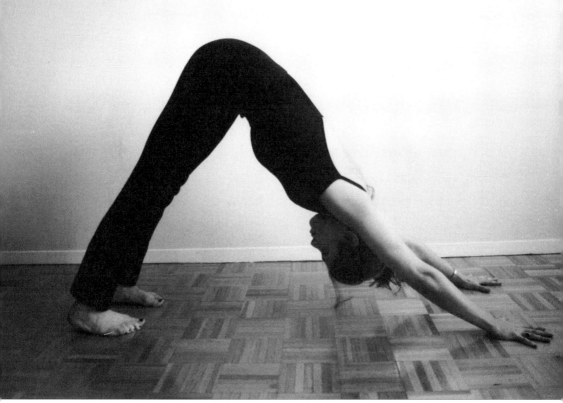

Downward Facing Dog

2. Try to hold your head up and stretch the spine. Remain here and take two deep breaths.

3. Exhale. Move the torso closer to the legs and rest the head on the knees. Stay here for a moment and inhale and exhale deeply.

4. Again, raise the head and look up while keeping your palms on the floor. After two breaths, inhale deeply and come back to Mountain Pose.

These are just a few of the *asanas* that help with illness and discomfort. You will certainly discover many new ones on your own. Like we discussed earlier, all the different aspects of yoga lead to the same place: union of body, mind, and heart. That union is total wellness.

Meditation is also an important part of the yoga experience because it helps to bring about that union. You probably never thought sitting still with your eyes closed could make you feel better. But in the next chapter, you'll learn that it can.

Chapter 6

Meditation

Have you ever stopped to look at waves crashing on the beach, or at a candle flame, or even a tree in the park, and felt as if you were lost in the image, as if you were entering a trance? You may not have realized it, but in a way, you were meditating at that moment.

Meditation is really just focusing intently on one sound, idea, image, or goal. Remember a few chapters ago, when we discussed how fast our society runs, with e-mail, cell phones, and TV as our constant companions? Well, practicing meditation is a way to prevent your world from spinning out of control. It's like going on vacation in your mind when you can't with your body.

A regular meditation practice can bring tremendous rewards. Do you ever have trouble concentrating on homework or simply reading a book? Do you feel as if you sometimes have to read the same paragraph over and over again? Meditation can bring you an inner peace that will help you master concentration. When you slow down to meditate once per day, or maybe a few times per week, the stuff that used to take forever to finish will come easier to you. Meditation will also help you to sleep better. If you meditate for a few minutes before you go to bed, you will wake up less tired and more refreshed. When your alarm clock rings or your mom yells at you to get out of bed, you will open your eyes ready to take on any challenge. You will also remember your dreams more easily.

Mantras

So how do we begin? The first task is to choose a *mantra*. A *mantra* is simply a sound, word, or phrase that is repeated over and over as you meditate. It can be spoken aloud as in chanting, or repeated silently to oneself in meditation.

A lot of people think the best *mantras* are the ones that have no clear meaning, the ones that are just sounds. This is so that the meditator will not get involved in *thinking* about meditation. This may sound a little confusing, but the point of meditation is to go beyond or underneath thought. You master your mind by controlling it.

A Catholic form of meditation, saying the rosary, is one kind of *mantra*. Because I am Jewish, I use a Hebrew prayer, "Ribbono Shel Olam," when I meditate;

it means "all one source." (Because Hebrew is not my first language, the phrase feels more like a sound than an idea.) You can choose whatever *mantra* you want. You can even repeat the word "love" over and over.

If you don't have any ideas for a *mantra,* I suggest using "hamsa." It works with the breath. You say "ham" (huh-ahhm) on the inhalation and "sa" on the exhalation. (*Hamsa* is an Arabic symbol that is said to protect people. It looks like a hand.)

Let's begin. The first thing you need to do is find a safe, quiet space in which to meditate. Never meditate in bed. Although meditation can sometimes make you fall asleep, sleeping and meditating are two separate activities.

The spot you chose for your *asana* practice might be a good place to meditate. You can light some incense or a scented candle. (*Nag Champa* is the most preferred incense in yoga circles.) Some people like to use a meditation cushion to sit on. It's not necessary, but you might want to sit on a pillow to feel more comfortable. (It's really important not to get caught up in your leg falling asleep as you meditate!) Sit in the Lotus pose or cross-legged. You can even sit against the wall or in a chair if you want back support.

Close your eyes. Breathe naturally. Try to sit for a minute or two before you begin repeating your *mantra* to slow down the breath and heart rate. Bring your attention to your breath. Do this gently, without force. Then begin to silently repeat "ham" on the inhale and

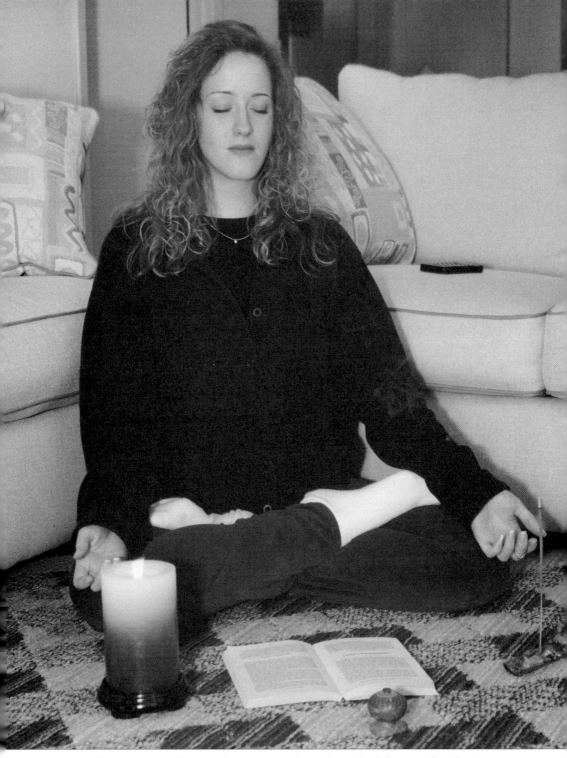

Incense, candles, and *mantras* clear the mind for meditation.

"sa" on the exhale (or whatever your chosen *mantra* is). Let yourself "melt" into the process.

Thoughts, even obsessive ones, are likely to come. Try to let them come and go without attachment. Imagine your thoughts dancing across the movie screen of your mind, but pretend that it really is a movie. Pretend that all the worries and fears that control you are someone else's movie. Note the thoughts, and don't try to change or control them. If you realize that you are thinking thoughts, gently move back into your *mantra*. This might happen every few seconds. Do not become frustrated. It's perfectly normal. Meditation is an art that takes lots of practice. Just give it time.

Meditation teachers suggest that one should meditate for at least twenty minutes per session. That is a good goal, but if you feel you can only do it for five or ten minutes at first that's okay, too. You can work your way up to longer periods of meditation. You may find yourself in a deep state of relaxation. You may not. You may not feel anything at first, because you are still so attached to your thoughts.

When you are finished, sit for a moment or two until you come back to normal awareness. Don't get up too fast. (It's okay to glance at a clock if you are timing your meditation. But don't use an alarm clock to shock you out of your altered state.)

There are different opinions regarding the best time to meditate. In the morning before breakfast or in the evening before dinner are both good times. (Digestion is known to shut down during meditation, so it's a good idea to have an empty stomach.)

The most important part of meditation is simply attempting to do it. The intention to meditate is more important than getting it "right" because there is no right way to do it. Just try it, and be with your *mantra*. You might fall asleep, or obsess, or try to plan your science project during meditation. Allow it to happen. Just gently go back to the *mantra*. Be patient; you will see results.

Chanting and *Bhakti*

Bhakti, *love of god, is the essence of all spiritual discipline . . . Through love one acquires renunciation and discrimination naturally.*

—Ramakrishna

Bhakti yoga is the path of love and devotion. It is different from romantic love. There is no possessiveness with *bhakti*. When you are "in love" with your boyfriend, for instance, and he forgets to call you, you might feel depressed and lonely. But the great thing about *bhakti* yoga is that you can have it whenever you want. It is inside of you.

Chanting, a form of meditation and practice of *bhakti* yoga, is performed aloud. Have you ever heard a song that suddenly made you cry? Maybe it was the melody,

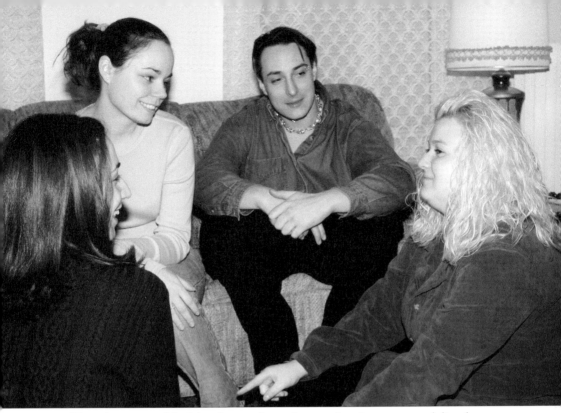

Hanging out with friends can be a form of *satsang,* or spiritual gathering.

or the lyrics. A *kirtan* is a kind of sing-along. The leader of the *kirtan* sings a verse, and the group repeats it. This is another way of calming the mind. The repetition is like the repeating of the *mantra.*

Two leaders of *kirtan* are Krishna Das (in New York) and Bhagavan Das (near San Francisco). They have both put out chanting records (listed in the resources section). Another name for gathering is *satsang. Satsang* is meeting at the feet of the wise. Every time you take a yoga class or go to a lecture you are at *satsang.* Even when you hang out with friends and learn from them, it is a form of *satsang.* It is yet another form of meditation. It helps you to focus the mind.

Divine Bliss

As you study yoga more extensively, you will learn more about who you really are. That is the central purpose of yoga. Right now, you might think that you *are* your body. Yoga will teach you that you are *not* your body—your body is a tool that you've been given to help you realize who you really are.

Yoga will show you that everyone on earth is connected, from your neighbors to your teachers to your parents to your favorite movie star. If we remember that *ahimsa* is the founding principle of yoga, and apply it in our lives, we will be teaching profoundly needed lessons to those around us.

All of the yoga paths described in this book lead to the same place: union of body, mind, and soul. Whether you choose to sing, meditate, do *asana* practice, or all of the above, you will find your own brand of bliss.

Glossary

ahimsa **(ah-HIM-sah)** Nonviolence, absolute compassion.

asana **(AH-sah-na)** A posture or seat. The third of the *sutras* of Patanjali.

ashtanga **yoga** The eight-limbed path of yoga developed by Patanjali.

bhakti **(BAK-tee) yoga** The yoga of devotion.

bindi A jewel worn over the third eye (on the forehead) to symbolize expanded consciousness.

guru **(GOO-roo)** A spiritual guide or teacher.

incense A type of spice that is often burned during spiritual ceremonies to create a sweet smell.

karma **(KAR-muh) yoga** Action and selfless service.

kirtan **(KUR-tan)** Singing or chanting.

mantra **(MAHN-tra)** A sound or phrase that is repeated to aid in meditation.

meditation The act of focusing, or getting to a higher state of consciousness by quieting the mind.

mulabhanda **(moo-lah-BAN-dah)** "Holding the root" of the body. A contraction of the area from the navel to the anus held during *asana* practice.

Namaste **(NA-ma-stay)** A greeting that means "I bow to the divine in you."

om (AUM) The all-pervading sound used in meditation and chanting.

Patanjali The ancient Indian sage who created the *Ashtanga* system of yoga.

prana **(PRAH-na)** Life energy.

pranayama **(prahn-ay-YAHM-uh)** Control of *prana* through breathing exercises.

sadhana **(sah-DAHN-ah)** A spiritual way or practice.

Sanskrit The ancient language of India.

satsang **(SATT-sang)** Sitting at the feet of the wise; gathering with other people on the path to further your practice.

sutra(s) **(SOO-trah)** Thread or verse. The Yoga Sutras of Patanjali were written over 5,000 years ago; they are the bible of yoga.

ujayii **(YOU-jie)** The type of *pranayama* used in *asana* practice: mouth closed, audible hissing sound at the back of the throat.

yama Restraint. The first of the eight limbs of Ashtanga yoga.

yoga Union with the divine.

Where to Go for Help

Because yoga has exploded in popularity over the past few years, there are many ways to get started. If you want to begin an *asana* or meditation practice, you can read more books or rent videos or attend classes.

First, go to your local library to see what books and videos you can borrow. Look in the yellow pages under yoga, fitness, or gyms. (Many gyms hold yoga classes every week. If they don't, tell them you would attend if they added yoga to the schedule!) Feel free to approach any yoga instructor after class and ask questions such as "Where did you do your training?" and "Do you teach anywhere else in town?" Also, petition your gym teachers at school to incorporate yoga into the curriculum.

If you can't find anyone doing yoga in your hometown, or you have chosen to do a solitary practice, look to local, alternative bookstores for help. Health food stores are another good source of information. If you want to listen to music made just for yoga practice, you should be able to find it at a local music store.

Most of the resources listed in this book can also be ordered from the Jivamukti Yoga Center, 404 Lafayette Street, Third Floor, New York, NY 10003; (800) 295-6814, extension 211. Ask for its catalog.

Books

The *Bhagavad Gita* is considered to be the best of Hindu texts, the Bible of Hinduism. You can read any good translation; ask your librarian or bookseller.

Das, Hari Baba. *Ashtanga Yoga Primer.* Santa Cruz: Sri Rama Publishing, 1981.

Iyengar, B.K.S. *Light on Yoga.* New York: Shocken Books, 1979.

Scaravelli, Vanda. *Awakening the Spine: The Stress-Free Yoga That Works with the Body to Restore Health, Vitality and Energy.* San Francisco: Harper San Francisco, 1995.

Yogananda, Parmahansa. *Autobiography of a Yogi.* Los Angeles: Self-Realization Fellowship, 1993.

World Wide Web/Internet Links

Any Web search will turn up thousands of links to yoga sites, but here is a sampling of some of the best resources:

Kripalu Center
http://www.vgernet.net/kali/entrance.html

Spirit Web Organization
http://www.spiritweb.org/Spirit/Yoga/Overview.html

Spirituality/Yoga Home Page
http://www.geocities.com/RodeoDrive/1415/index.html

Yoga Internet Resources
http://www.holisticmed.com/www/yoga.html

Magazines
Yoga Journal
For subscription information:
(800) 600-YOGA

Videography
What Is Yoga?
(800) 295-6814
Available from Jivamukti, this is a great introduction to
the philosophy and practice of yoga. It is not an *asana*
practice videotape.

Yoga Journal's Yoga Practice for Beginners
(800) 254-8464
Web site: http://www.livingarts.com
The entire *Yoga Journal* series of videotapes from
Healing Arts Publishing is excellent. You can order
from the Living Arts catalog or visit its Web site.

Yoga with Richard Freeman Ashtanga Yoga, The Primary Series
(888) 398-YOGA
This tape is for advanced students.

Discography
Alice Coltrane, *Divine Songs, Glorious Chants*
Sanskrit chanting set to gospel/jazz rhythms.

Bhagavan Das, *In Concert, Mt. Vision*
> Available on cassette only, through the
> Hanuman Foundation.

Krishna Das, *One Track Heart, Pilgrim Heart*

Jim Donovan, *Indigo*
> Jim Donovan is the drummer for the band
> Rusted Root. This CD uses repetition of the
> sacred sound "om" and creates an awesome
> setting for meditation.

Ravi Shankhar, *The Sounds of India*
> A great introduction to Indian classical music.

Index

About the Author

Stefanie Iris Weiss has been practicing yoga since 1993. She is a teacher and writer living in New York City.

Photo Credits

Cover photo by Brian T. Silak. P. 8 © Everett Collection; pp. 10, 14 © Archive Photos; pp. 17, 18, 22, 28, 52, 55 by Brian T. Silak. All other photos by Karen Tom.